A Journey To The Centre Of My Heart

'An inspiring Cardiac Revelations, And
Total Body Rejuvenation'.

Ray Funns

EXPRESSION OF APPRECIATION

I would like to express our wholehearted appreciation specifically:
To the NHS, for providing such first-class Resource towards my personal health care without which this journey would not have been possible.
To The NHS staff of the Cardiology dept. on the Tower Block of the North Middlesex Hospital in North London UK and the Heart Hospital in Westmoreland Street W1., for their contribution in helping me find solutions
And finally To my Doctor at the Latymer Road Surgery. Enfield UK. Who worked tirelessly to insure that I overcome my health problem.

The Journey' Author and Editor
FunnCh Publishing

Ray Funns

Disclaimer

Prologue

I have undertaken the task of bringing my health problems to Kindle and to the public via my online video Portal. I have taken on the responsibility of finding out why my body is in this mess and an effort to understand my health problems, why I got it, its physical effects on me ant how I can get rid of it.

Having undergone such scary medical journey, I was determined to write about it and about other health problems that may affect me and my family. As a search enthusiast, I will use my search expertise to source medical solutions which would easily be understandable to a layman like me. These would be compiled within my free health video Channel to be released online so that people can view and learn from it. This portal would be totally transparent, meaning that it would be interactive, enabling visitors to make valued contributions and even send in videos of any health solutions they would wish to *share*.

When this portal is ready, readers of this health publication will have automatic access. This video portal would serve as a surprise Bonus for acquiring this first publication and other subsequent health investigations that will follow. An access detail for my Personal health video portal is clearly available in this Report. I hope that as you read on, you will find this brief medical journey inspiring too.

Contents

A Journey to the Centre of My Heart

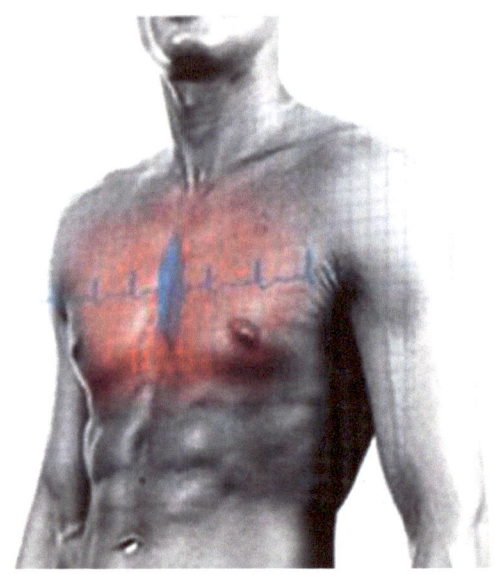

Image1 - Zone Of Pain From Reflux

Introduction

This is a true story of how my system suffered and how I was determined to find the root of my problem. I never set out to write a book on medical matters because I am not a doctor or any form of medical authority, however, I realised it would help a few people who may be experiencing the same problem that I had, I was motivated to write down this journey because I got my system completely cleaned or rejuvenated. I hope that by telling my story, you would learn from my experience…

My name is Ray. I started getting worried when I realized a constant burning in my chest sometimes whenever I eat something. I tried to see if I can get rid of this heartburning sensation in my chest with over-the-counter drugs such as Alka Zelter, Epsom Salt and some other heartburn recommendation. At this point in time I didn't really think I needed a doctor's advice for what I feel is a common problem. But as the problem persisted, I made up my mind to see my doctor about it.

The outcome of my visit to my doctor and the advice I received was the main motivating factor that pushed me into a journey to discover my inside. The project was so successful because it gave me the opportunity to find out for myself the best and the most natural and secure way to forever rid oneself of this truly uncomfortable body malfunction called Heartburn.

In addition to uncovering this, I was able to discover how every part of the body is tied together, especially the causes and effects of problems that will affect the heart, and consequently the whole body function. My best discovery while taking on this task is a comprehensive publication called *'Heartburn No More'* researched and produced by Jeff Martins. It is what finally enabled me to rid myself of heartburn permanently'. But initially when I went to see my doctor about my problem, something else other that heartburn was diagnosed. It was scary! This REPORT is a concise detail of what I went through in my quest to find out what was wrong. It is an eye opener for me which eventually led me to the discovery of the best cure for heartburn and a complete heart and system clean-up

A Journey to the Centre of My Heart

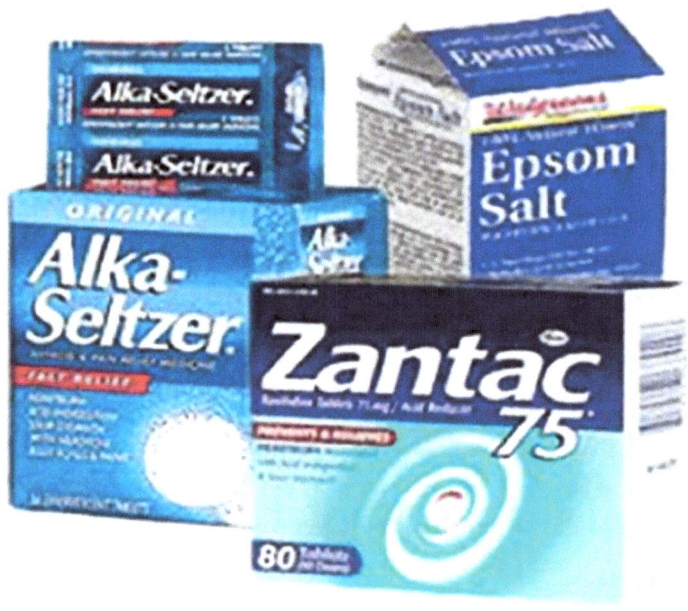

Image2 – Over The Counter Medication

Smoking and my persistent pain

What Made My Situation Scary?

What really made the situation scary for me is that I went to one of my Nigerian family friends one evening and after having a meal of pounded yam and codfish stew, which was really a very delicious but hot West African meal, I felt as though I had over-eaten. My stomach seemed much heavier than normal, and I can feel my chest really burning and heavy. I was expecting to have the usual hiccup, burping or belching which usually come up on me when I eat or swallow, because although I was worried about their frequency of occurrence, I do sometimes feel relieved when they come up, especially if I ate a lot. But the expected belch never came and I felt as if I have trapped wind inside my chest. As I left my friends home to walk across to get into the car, my whole body felt so weak due to the burning and heaviness on my chest, and my legs became very heavy too.

Early Signs of Problems

I began to really get worried way back in 2010 when I suddenly started having instant hiccup every time I swallow food. Although I have always had hiccup from my childhood days, I always thought it to be natural body function that's common to all humans. But from the above date, I began to notice hiccups and burping coming up on me mostly when I swallow. As I began to think more about what could be the reason for this experience, what was always on my mind was that I am having this problem because of my **20 cigarettes a day habit**. I wished I could stop smoking, but the problem is that I really honestly enjoy this horrible habit, and find it hard to break, despite the fact that I usually experienced a certain burning feeling just right under my breast. It wasn't a situation that got me immensely worried because it only lasted for a few minutes.

But I did begin to dwell on it more... Friends were advising me... Oh! Just go to the chemist and get some ***antacid solutions*** and follow the directives and that would get rid of your problem. I did take their advice and even had to get some heartburn cures recommended by the pharmacist at the chemist. Yet my problem continued. By 2011 my symptom became more prevalent, and I started to resort to some medication through my doctor. I had used one called Prevacid. On some occasions I have used Alka-Seltzer, Zantac and Epsom Salt

North Midd Experience – The Journey

My Doctor's Preliminary Diagnosis

I did manage to drive home, and in the morning, I went to my doctor, and a preliminary diagnosis from my doctor suggested that I have a **heart condition**, and was placed on medication. My doctor being such a good man, nervous and being always very concerned with my health decided to send me to North Middlesex Hospital cardiology department in London UK, to have my chest examined. It wasn't as straightforward as it seemed because from the moment of my preliminary diagnosis, I went to pieces and became so damned worried about my health. Some members of my family also became so worried for me, because if the doctor thinks that I have a heart condition, it must be true. It took about six months before I received a medical appointment at the north Middlesex Hospital.

How My Journey Began

The first appointment was simply an initial explanation of the protocols and procedures involved prior to actually lying onto the examination table. During this initial meeting, I was surprised to notice that there were about 8 people in a queue also waiting

to be interviewed. I thought I was the only one with a problem. It was a long wait before my turn came up. When it did, I was welcomed quite friendly, and I accepted apologies for having to wait so long. As I was seated down, my mind was curious as I don't know what bad news I am going to hear.

A Journey to the Centre of My Heart

'We invited you to come today so that we may familiarise you with procedures and the protocols prior to your examination.. It is possible that you have a heart condition. We cannot be sure until you undergo a heart examination'.

The cardiologist went on to explain the procedure involved…. After that I was handed a piece of paper containing questionnaires I must complete and sign before continuing the interview. There are some sections that explained the risk I am going to take which mentioned statistics of how many lost their life during the actual procedure that I am about to undergo.

Just to be aware of what is involved I was to be taken to the theatre to undergo what is termed Cardiac Catherisation or coronary angiogram where a dye is pumped through the groin into the arteries that carries blood to and from the heart, and through x-ray cardiologists are able to detect any problem in the

heart. This was explained to me and they would not go ahead with the procedure unless I sign and date that piece of questionnaire paper handed to me. I did sign it and they went on to tell me how this was going to be done and what I should have with me during the examination and what I must not eat before the operation. They will write me and let know the date for the operation. I kept this appointment eventually, and after going through the admission protocols I was ushered into the *Coronary Angiography* room and was asked for permission to allow medical students to gather round my naked body, and watch procedures as part of their learning experience. Oh! Well whatever! Hiding my nudity is not really important to me this time. I don't mind as long as I wouldn't experience a lot of pain or die in the process.

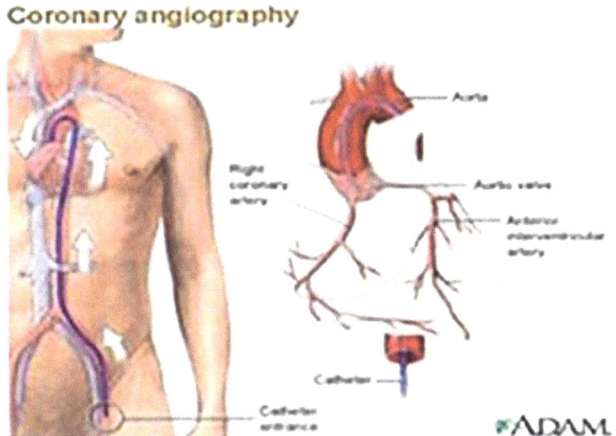

Coronary angiography is performed to detect obstruction in the coronary arteries of the heart. During the procedure a catheter (thin flexible tube) is inserted into an artery in your arm or groin and then threaded carefully into the heart. The blood vessels of the heart are then studied by injection of contrast media through the catheter. A rapid succession of X-rays (fluoroscopy) is taken to view blood flow.

Image3 - Diagram Showing Coronary Angiography

I was to undergo coronary angiogram, and was advised to lie on my back, and if I want, I can watch the whole procedure on screen hanging right in front of me. The effect of the anaesthetic I was given made me feel quite dazed. However, I could notice a tube being inserted on my groin as I was told I can watch the screen and observe how the dye travels through my body via the arteries towards my heart. It was so surreal that I could feel as if I was actually travelling and walking right through towards the centre of my heart.

Gripped by my Fears

Really Scared for My Life...

I was really scared because trying to overcome my heartburn problem seems to have led to the discovery of something more serious within my system. After my examination, I was summoned by the cardiologist eventually, and was told that I had mild atheroma of coronary arteries, but free from any significant heart disease. What on earth is **atheroma of coronary arteries**?

What this means according to the cardiologist is that there is evidence of an early stage of the hardening *of plaque deposits within the walls of the arteries in my heart, such that if unchecked could build up into* **angina***. This could be real disaster for me!* The outcome of the hospital visit was that I was to be referred to the Heart Hospital for further examination possibly Magnetic Resonance Imaging (MRI). More bad news! Meanwhile, I was prescribed extra medications to clear these deposits from my newly discovered health problem. Now because this is a heart-related problem, it had grave consequences for my lifestyle.

My Visit to the Heart Hospital:

It was again a long wait before I received another appointment to go to the Heart Hospital for further scan because the one carried out at the North Midd was inconclusive. As I went there it was exactly the same procedure as happened at North Middlesex. And to cut the story shorter, I was to lie on my back and be rolled inside this huge drum armed with a huge ear plugged headphone with a mouthpiece for instant communication with the operators on the outside, in case I was to experience any sudden discomfort, I was also equipped with a button to press for emergency.

With a feeling of being inside a coffin, some strange thoughts did go through my mind, like what would I do if there was an unexpected power failure, all those fears coupled with the continuous background noise of the scanner, made me feel a bit scared for my life, but overall the machine was painless and soothingly comfortable with just the right temperature. At last after lying there for approximately 25 minutes, the door opened and I had to put my clothes back on, and was free to leave. The result according to the specialists would be made available to my doctor within a couple of weeks.

Before I left I was curious to know more, so I asked the cardiologist if he could briefly explain if I should be worried about my heart, and he went on to show me few problems that can confront the heart. The Cardiologists produced some images identical to the images shown below that enabled me to understand the delicate nature of the heart. *'You have to understand that any minute obstruction to the natural flow of blood inside the arteries which carries blood to the heart has a significant effect on the overall energy level of the body'*, he said.

So if one is always feeling weak and constantly tired, this indicates that the natural flow is being compromised somewhere within because the heart is solely responsible for supplying specific and constant amount to all parts, therefore when these deposits start to clog up the walls of the arteries, if left unchecked would eventually build up and become really difficult to remove and would eventually affect the body's energy level.

A Journey to the Centre of My Heart

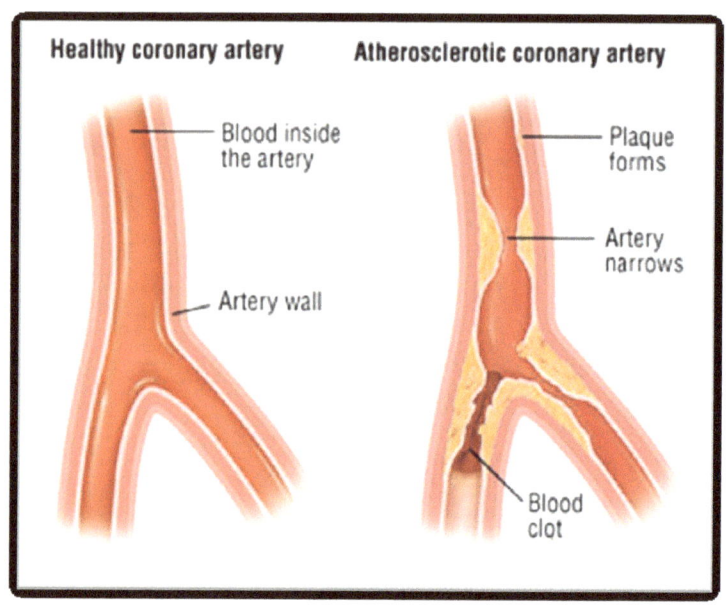

Image 4 - Showing clean and defective arteries

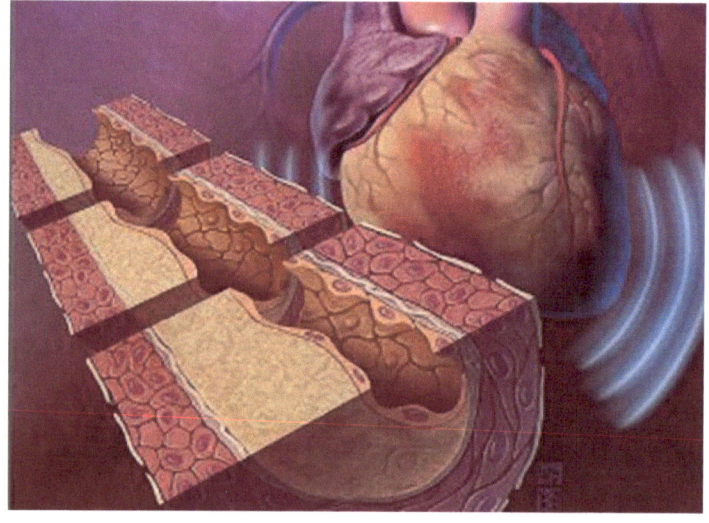

Image 5 - Showing cut-away section of severely clogged arteries

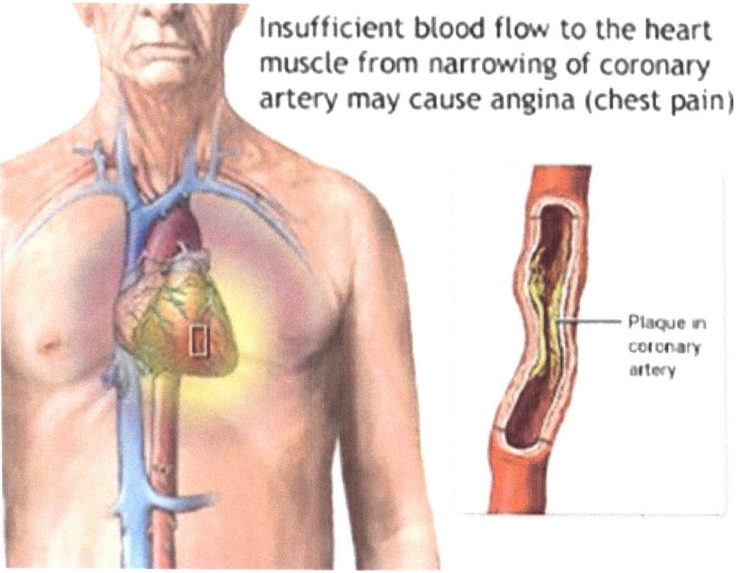

Insufficient blood flow to the heart muscle from narrowing of coronary artery may cause angina (chest pain)

Plaque in coronary artery

Image 6 - More example of deposits

This is the main reason why the body lack energy to function naturally., To be fit, strong, and athletic, the Heart must be free of the harmful substances we ignorantly subject it to like smoking drug taking and high cholesterol foods, the cardiologist explained.

Images that killed My Smoking Habit

The scariest and the most shocking images I saw during these visits was the effect of smoking on the lungs. After seeing these, the First and foremost thing to do is that I definitely

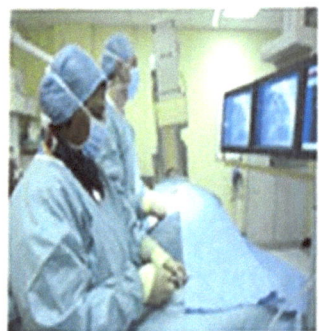 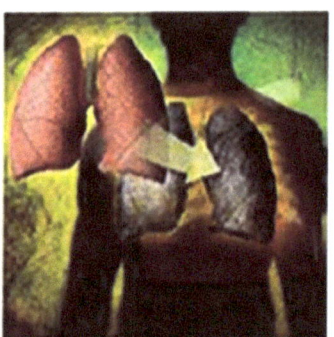

Image 7 – Left: operations theatre.| Right: smoker's lungs

must give up smoking! Period, because according to the specialists, this could have been the main culprit, coupled with high cholesterol diets, these definitely contribute to other problems such as cancer, lung and kidney problems too. In fact all of these can be a direct result of extensive smoking alone.

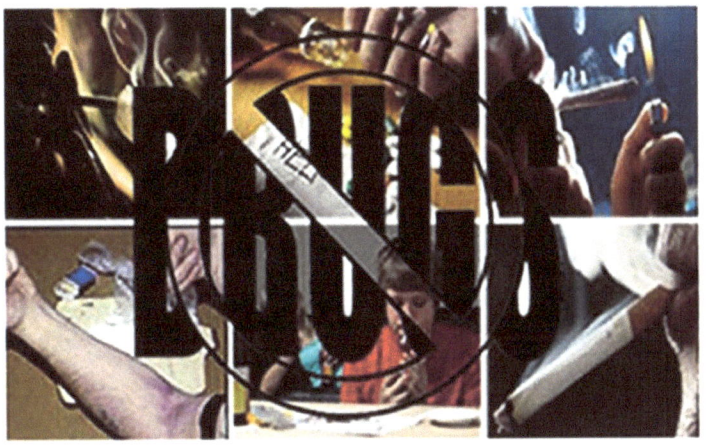

Image8 - No To Smoking and Drugs

I finally Gave Up Smoking

The persistent use of drugs like cocaine, heroin, and marijuana and of course cigarettes is mostly to blame for those deposits on the arteries. He explained. As for myself, I don't do drugs like cocaine, heroin, and marijuana, but I only smoke cigarettes. So in my case, heavy smoking must be blamed for those deposits. Well... Finally it had to be done. I finally, gave up smoking, and how I managed to do this will be the subject I would write about in future

My Doctor Warns!

"You definitely must start eating a lot of vegetables from now onwards"... My doctor warned, and went to great length of telling me the importance of having dominant fruit and vegetable diet –

'They are loaded with minerals, vitamins, phytonutrients, fibre, and antioxidants. He said. They help to get rid of those deposits and a number of chronic problems including obesity, cancer, diabetes, and **heartburn** *and* **heart disease**. *Alongside, they are great for better digestion. And the Anti-oxidants present in fruits and vegetables fight a number of diseases. They also tackle free radicals that are very harmful to the body'*

Point taken... So much so that nowadays my kitchen and dining table is littered with varying types of fruits and vegetables, and I have sort of got used to this form of dieting, and it is good. What about the main condition which led me to come to the hospital in the first place, which is my heartburn problem.

My persistent heartburn

Well! Even though I went through all these trouble, the medication I was taking for my heartburn as described earlier still wasn't doing the business; instead I was still having a bit of heartburn, coupled with some adverse side effects on me, due probably to the additional medication which I was assigned to, to help to clear the deposits on the walls of my arteries,

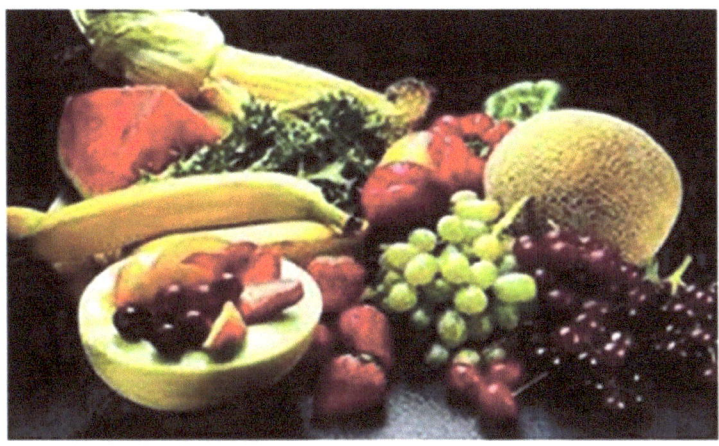

Image 9 – Healthy Foods For The Heart

After taking these medications for a while, It was making my legs too tired and I get the feeling as if my legs are turning to jelly when I walk. This side effects situation improved when my doctor reduced the dosage of one of the tablets I was prescribed. But... My original problem was still there

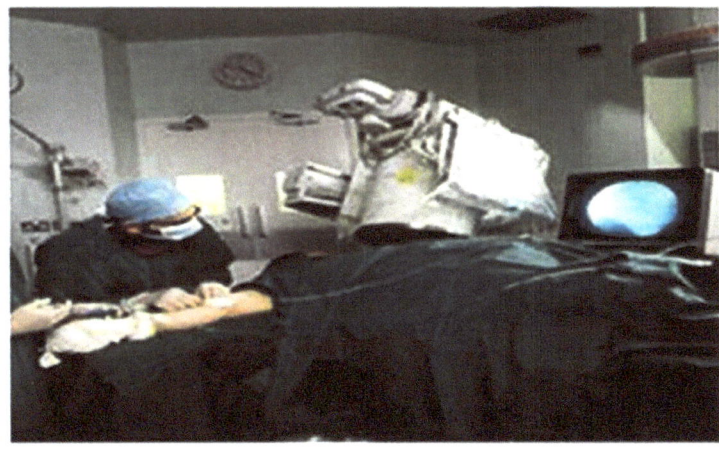

A Journey to the Centre of My Heart

However, I did manage to find a solution, not by any form of medication, but through sustained research to find out all I can because everyone I describe my problem to told me I have heartburn... Heartburn! That doesn't seem to go away, even with all the medication? It was only by chance that I had the answer to this problem.

Heartburn cure out of the blue

At Last a Solution for My Heartburn

I couldn't quite recollect the exact date in 2011 when I opened my laptop and typed in '*heartburn remedy*' on Google's search box, and was presented with a number of websites. The one that was quite prominent was 'Heartburn No More™'. Well I didn't even bother to look at it because there were other more prominent ones also... However, after about a few weeks going through one site after another trying to find the one I can trust to solve my problem, a friend emailed me a specific recommendation I must try - a scientifically arranged and professionally presented step-by-step daily planned dietry instructions on how to rejuvenate and get rid of heartburn and many other forms of ABDOMINAL problems in any body.

It turned out to be the same 'Heartburn No More' I previously overlooked. So, I immediately bought the information Pack and followed up the instructions. I would describe it as a sort of carefully organised DIY at home detox or rehab plan, for anyone who haven't got the kind money needed to go to those highly expensive health and body rejuvenation or Rehab centres now available in major cities.

Within two weeks of trying it, I could feel as if I was morphing into a new fresh form. The hiccup, the belching, and burping all gone. That constant chest pain and tiredness disappeared. My legs became sharper; I can now run quite a distance without getting tired.

I still do not know if what I had was heartburn, because the doctors did not diagnose heartburn. However, as I desperately followed the directives on this '*Heartburn No More*' pack, I started to feel better and different.

A Journey to the Centre of My Heart

Happy To Be On a Mission

I am happy to be on this mission right now and to let people know about this fantastic Information pack. Please if you have used it and know about it give us a feedback at

mailto:rayfunnsinfo@gmail.com *and let me know about your experience and how you feel and how we can help others...* As I got my heartburn sorted, I thought it would be a good idea to use my experience to alert people about the fragile nature of the body.

While I was in the hospital, I was hearing about so many depressing health terms relating to the heart, angina, gerd, heart attack, congestive heart failure, lung transplant, Constipation, Abdominal problems, to name but just a few, so I decided… well I will lose nothing to have first-hand knowledge of these terms. Hence I made up my mind to embark on a convenient research in my own unique way to discover for myself what some of the terms mean and how they might affect me, and if there are some precautions that can be taken to avoid these in future

My Health Report

My New Idea to Alert Others

Now, here's the thing, the experience that I went through as a result of Heartburn opened a great door for me. So much so that I decided that it would be a great idea from a layman's point of view to document every health problem that has troubled me all my life, and seek to find answers to those problems.

I am not going to research every personal health problem, except those that affect me and my family. We have had a lot of medical issues over the years, and I believe that out there, there may be others who may be having the same problems we had or may have in future, so I thought to myself.. Why not use the skills you have as a CAD technician, Mini-Site Designer and an accomplished online Video Producer.... to bring some medical problems and solutions on screen so that others can learn and benefit from my experience too and maybe discover few things that can help the body.

It is true that I can produce original videos on any subject, but what are not at my disposal are logistics, expertise and finance, so instead I have opted to use the current social media resources which is freely available online. I came up with the idea of using the vast resources available to us especially YouTube Videos to provide specific health information platform that would be free to use.

Although I am a video producer, I don't really have to start producing original videos on medical issues that I know nothing about. Huge thanks to YouTube **'Share'** facility, my idea right now is to go online and source some significant problems solving health videos in varying medical fields. And those problems will only be the ones that my family and I suffered and the ones that may affect us in the future, most of which can be avoided by understanding them. I believe people would benefit from this humble free resource

We Are All Guilty

We are all guilty of taking our health for granted, and what most people don't get is that there are those of us who go to sleep at night and never wake up again in the morning... They are dead... gone too soon! Possibly, as a result of some neglected health problems. **Therefore we must take steps to look after our bodies.** We all talk about creating wealth and being happy... these cannot be accomplished unless you have good health... **so really the body comes first**.

Instant Access to my Online Health Video Platform

Yes! I have become hugely motivated into going this route after the experience from my journey in hospital... I am going to concentrate in sourcing health issues and remedies that I personally encountered, and bring my findings out to those who may learn from it.

I am in the process of completing my first health Information Platform which will be in Video Format, showing information about the Heart and various problems associated with it. If you had this report you are reading, *you would automatically have instant access to my Personal Health Video Platform indefinitely* Free access to this facility is my planned THANK YOU Bonus for getting this first issue... You have permanent access! ENJOY it whenever you can!

My Platform is not yet ready but if you are interested simply send me a blank email right now with a subject-line – '**Personal Health Video Channel**' to :mailto:rayfunnsinfo@gmail.com Your blank email would automatically enter the ***Personal Health***

Video Channel List, and you will be given instant access ASAP once the platform is ready

Conclusion

Here's a quick summary about the Bits I discovered regarding the Heart and Heartburn!

Quick Summary

Chest pain is obviously the main reasons a person goes to the emergency room. While many maybe suffering from a heart attack, some actually may be experiencing **severe heartburn from abdominal troubles**. Sometimes, the pain caused by a heart attack and pain due to a severe heartburn episode is so difficult to distinguish that sophisticated medical testing is needed to determine whether or not one is having a **heart attack**. To make matters even more complicated, the two problems have many of the same symptoms and occur in similar types of people (For example, older people and people who are overweight).

The Heartburn pain I experienced includes:

A sharp, burning sensation just below the breastbone or ribs. Signs that is more typical of heart attack or angina (a severe pain in chest area) according to the doctors.

A feeling of tightness, or pain generally in the centre of the chest.

Sudden chest pain or pressure that worsens.

Dizziness,

Pain that sometimes spread to the shoulders, neck, jaw or arms.

Shortness of breath, often accompanied by a possible cold sweat.

If you ever experience similar pains that last for more than a few minutes or any warning signs of a heart attack, it is a good advice to seek immediate medical attention. If there's any confusion about whether your symptoms are *heartburn* or *a heart attack*, also seek immediate medical attention.

How I managed to give up smoking I loved so much'… to me is totally unbelievable. **I honestly did quit smoking**! I cannot say I regret the journey I took to find out what was wrong with me, because obviously I had Heartburn, which has been cleared! … Thanks to **Heartburn No More™**. But I also discovered that my system **was developing a mild sign of angina**

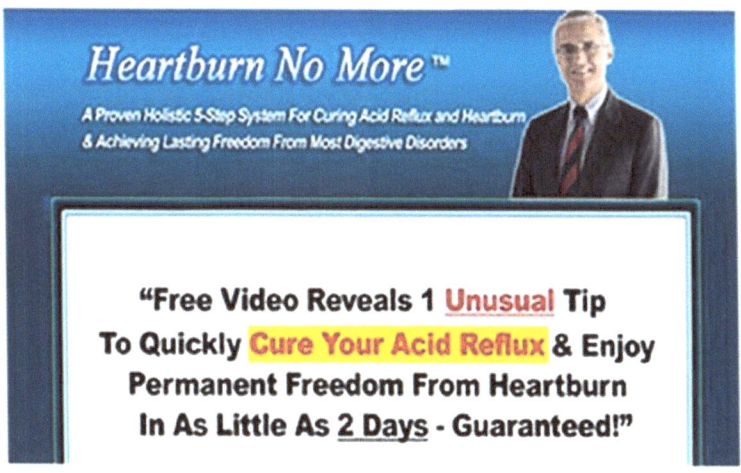

Image 11 – Heartburn No More Site

The Positive Effects of My Journey.

Without undertaking this journey I may not have discovered that problem which is now being resolved. **I am done with smoking for the rest of my life**. If you do smoke I must encourage you to quit. Initially it would almost seem unrealistic and even impossible to you because you think that you really enjoy it and it helps you deal with everyday stress. That's what I use to say to myself too. But!.. **Believe me you will be so happy that you managed to achieve the impossible. You will be full of life; you will smell fresh and have a lot more money in your pocket**. When I look back, I wished I never put that single stick of cigarette between my lips that resulted in my addiction to

nicotine. I may have wasted my hard earned cash all these years buying something that was gradually killing my body, but right now I am really happy that I was able to quit smoking and never to touch it ever again!.. Believe me... **Quitting is seriously empowering!**

I plan to make this manual widely available worldwide to make people aware of the danger in taking the Heart for granted. To make this possible I plan to create three more titles giving more in-depth consequences of neglect and lack of care for our bodies…these would serve as direct upgrades to this original. These would help spread this alert even further.

1. *"A Journey To The Centre Of My Heart"* *Body rejuvenation Classic Vol 1- This is my first health publication..*

2. *"A Paradise for Smoke Quitters"* - *Body rejuvenation Classic Vol 2 by R Funns*

3. *"Body And Smoke"* – *Body and soul rejuvenation Classic Vol 3 by R Funns*

4 *"The Engine Of Your Mind"*- *Body and soul rejuvenation Classic Vol 4 By R Funns*

Ray Funns

The next three Titles will be published individually as soon as they are ready. So please watch out for more.

I hope this helps!

Ray Funns

Recommendations

Simply scan with your mobile phone and gain instant access to Jeff Martins '*Heartburn No More*'

Image 12 – Barcode For HNM...Scan Image

About the Author

Ray funns is a co-founder of Netwealthcreations, and FunnCh Publishing. He works privately as a mobile optimised mini-site developer, and online video creator, a search expert and has recently discovered self-Publishing using Kindle. He suffered a heart situation that was inconclusively diagnosed. In his first kindle issue, Ray produced a precise true account of his journey to discover his health problems which he hopes others would learn from.

He has been an anonymous contributor to the Charities, and would like to further fund the **Heart foundation** *and the* **Sickle Cell** *charities from the sale of his kindle works. Ray now plans to make this manual widely available to make people aware of the dangers in taking the Body, especially the Heart for granted.*

To make this possible Ray is planning to publish three more titles as an upgrade to this original idea by bringing a layman's perspective to dangers affecting the body and possible solutions. This would help spread the alert further

Ray *is now completely free from this painful condition, and has this advice!*

'If you have any chest pains or heart-related problem such as Abdominal issues, **Heartburn** *or* **Acid Reflux***, or you are always feeling tired at home or at work, it maybe that your system need complete overhaul. You may not need a stressful journey to the hospital like I did, or contemplate spending thousands of cash on Rehab clinic. Simply type in* http://tinyurl.com/stop-hburn *into your browser for immediate access to Jeff Martins..* *"Heartburn No More™"* *It's a process that would* **enable your body to be completely rejuvenated'..**
-Ray Funns -

Appendices

Appendix1

Below are minimised screenshot of events and exact date
Brochure and location during my trip to North Middlesex
Hospital London Edmonton London N18

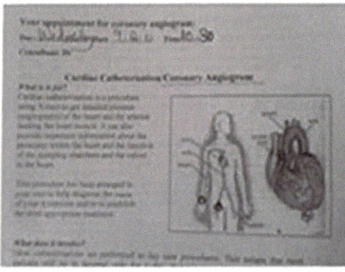

Appointment date 09/02/2011 at 10.30am.
This was the first interview stage.

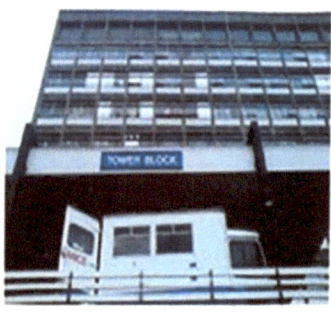

Tower Block at North Mid where scan
was carried out at the 8th floor.

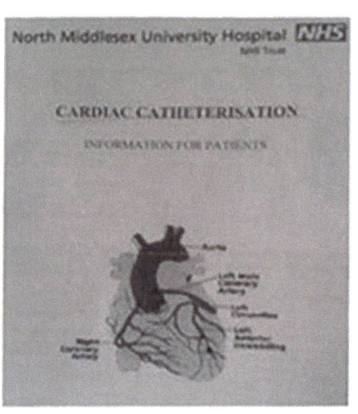

Scanned image of front cover of original
Information Brochure

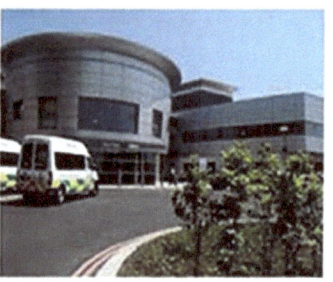

Main entrance at North Mid Hospital

Image 13 - Appointment - North-Middlesex Hospital

Ray Funns

Showing Heart Hospital appointment details

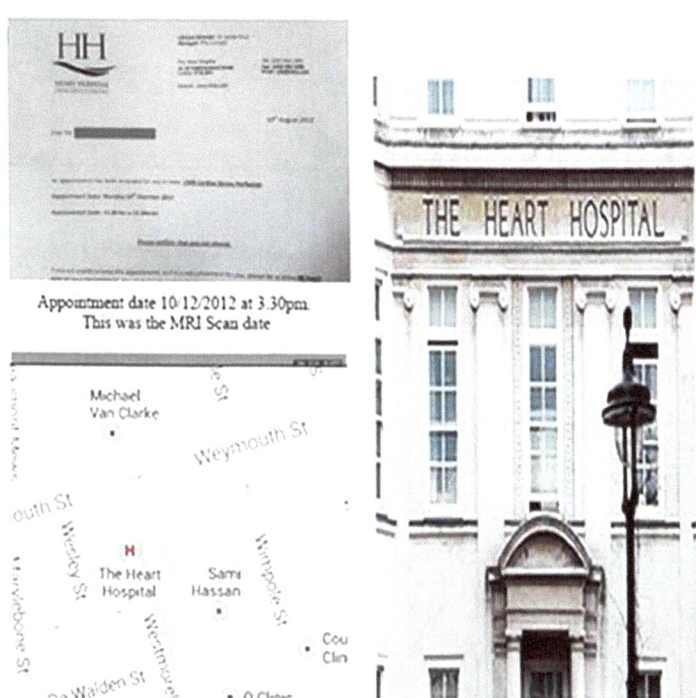

Appointment date 10/12/2012 at 3.30pm.
This was the MRI Scan date

Scanned image of front cover of original
street map inside Information Brochure

Clipped image of Main entrance
at the Heart Hospital in Westmoreland
Street W1

Image 14 - Appointment – The Heart Hospital London W1

A Journey to the Centre of My Heart

Appendix3

Screenshot Showing A friends Email recommending
Heartburn Product

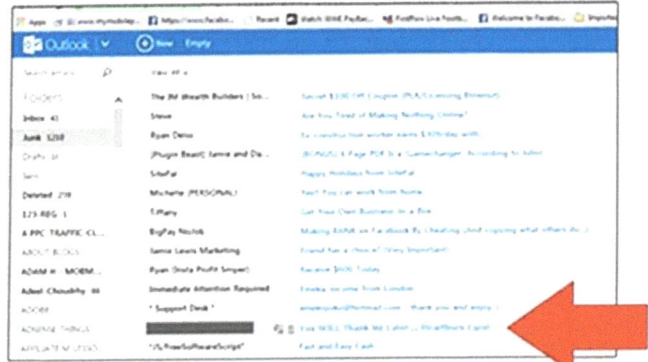

Screenshot of Inbox: red arrow showing email of Heartburn
Info shown below.

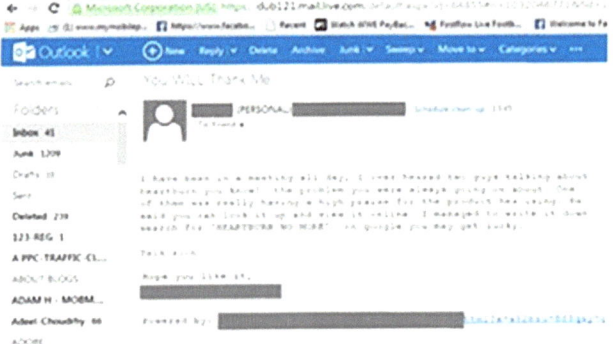

Screenshot of friend's email endorsing Heartburn Product

Image 15 – Heartburn Cure email

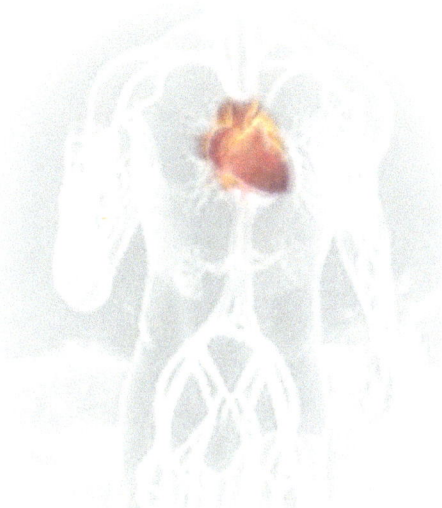

Funns, R, ' *A Journey To The Center Of My Heart',* **Edmonton Enfield: London.** Copyright© 2013 – FunnCh Publishing. All Rights Reserved

A Journey to the Centre of My Heart

Notes 1

Ray Funns

Notes 2

Notes 3